Dr. Miriam J. Johnson

The Hidden Health Code: Unlocking the Secrets to Vitality

Table of contents

The Science of Optimal Health: Separating Fact from Fiction

"The Science of Optimal Health: Separating Fact from Fiction" is to provide readers with an understanding of the current scientific evidence surrounding health and wellness. In this chapter, readers will learn to differentiate between what is based on solid scientific research versus what is simply a popular myth or fad.

It's begins by examining common myths that people believe about health, such as the idea that taking vitamins or supplements can replace a healthy diet. It's then delves into the latest scientific research on topics such as nutrition, exercise, sleep, stress, and mental health. It provides evidence-based recommendations on how readers can optimize their health based on this research.

Individuals are encouraged to be critical of health information they come across, especially on social media, and to seek out reliable sources backed by scientific evidence. The chapter also discusses the importance of consulting with a healthcare provider before making any major changes to one's lifestyle or diet.

It is important to have a solid understanding of what the latest scientific research says about the foundations of optimal health, and will be better equipped to make informed decisions about their own health and wellness.

For example, discusses the importance of a balanced and varied diet, based on whole foods, and recommends avoiding fad diets that promise quick results. It also explains the benefits of regular physical activity, including both cardio and strength training, and how even small amounts of movement throughout the day can improve overall health.

Additionally, discusses the importance of sleep and how inadequate sleep can have negative effects on physical and mental health. It also covers the effects of chronic stress on the body and mind, and provides strategies for managing stress and improving mental health. It is importance of seeking out reliable sources of health make their products appear healthier than they actually are, and provides tips on how to avoid falling for these tricks.

The chapter also discusses the benefits of meal planning and provides suggestions for quick and healthy meals that can be made at home. It emphasizes the importance of taking time to plan meals and snacks in advance, and provides strategies for making healthy choices when eating out.

One of the key strategies discussed in the chapter is the importance of reading food labels. The chapter provides guidance on how to read food labels in order to identify the most important information, such as serving size, calorie count, and nutrient content. It also discusses how to identify foods that are high in added sugars, sodium, and unhealthy fats.

The chapter emphasizes the importance of choosing whole, nutrient-dense foods over highly processed foods. It provides tips on how to shop for fresh produce, lean proteins, and healthy fats, and how to incorporate these ingredients into meals and snacks.

To help readers make healthy choices when eating out, the chapter also provides tips on how to order at restaurants, including how to navigate menus, identify healthy options, and make substitutions to make meals healthier.

Throughout the chapter, the emphasis is on taking a balanced and practical approach to nutrition. Readers are encouraged to make small, sustainable changes over time, rather than attempting extreme or restrictive diets that are difficult to maintain. The chapter also discusses the importance of taking time to plan meals and snacks in advance, and provides suggestions for quick and healthy meals that can be made at home.

Cracking the Code: Understanding Your Unique Health Needs

Cracking the Code: Understanding Your Unique Health, it is designed to help readers understand that health is not a one-size-fits-all solution, and that everyone has unique health needs that require a personalized approach. The chapter begins by introducing the concept of personalized medicine and the importance of understanding one's unique health needs.

There are different factors that can impact an individual's health, such as genetics, lifestyle, and environment. It explains how each of these factors can influence health outcomes and provides examples of how to modify each factor to improve health.

It is important toidentifying one's individual health needs and creating a personalized health plan. It provides guidance on how to identify areas of health that may require attention, such as nutrition, exercise, stress management, and sleep, and how to create a plan that addresses each area.

In addition, the chapter provides practical guidance on how to monitor one's health progress and adjust the health plan as needed. It explains the importance of tracking key health indicators, such as blood pressure, cholesterol levels, and blood sugar, and provides suggestions on how to track these indicators at home. Readers are encouraged to take an active role in their health and to prioritize self-care.

In summary, "Cracking the Code: Understanding Your Unique Health Needs" chapter provides readers with practical tips and tools for understanding their individual health needs and creating a personalized health plan. It emphasizes the importance of a personalized approach to health and provides guidance on how to monitor and adjust one's plan as needed.

The Role of Sleep in Health and Vitality

It begins by discussing the different stages of sleep and the importance of each stage in promoting restorative processes in the body. It explains how sleep impacts various aspects of health, including immune function, cognitive function, and emotional wellbeing.

There are factors that can interfere with quality sleep, such as stress, poor sleep habits, and medical conditions. It provides practical guidance on how to create a sleep-friendly environment and establish healthy sleep habits that can promote better quality sleep.

The health consequences of poor sleep, including increased risk for chronic diseases such as obesity, diabetes, and cardiovascular disease. It provides evidence-based information on how sleep disturbances can affect metabolic function, immune function, and cognitive function, and provides suggestions on how to improve sleep quality to reduce these risks.

The chapter provides readers with a deep understanding of the crucial role that sleep plays in maintaining optimal health and vitality. It explains how sleep is essential for the proper functioning of various bodily systems, including the immune system, cardiovascular system, and nervous system.

There are different stages of sleep, including non-rapid eye movement (NREM) and rapid eye movement (REM) sleep, and how each stage plays a vital role in promoting physical and mental restoration. It also discusses the importance of sleep quantity and quality, highlighting that adults typically need 7-9 hours of sleep per night.

Moreover, the chapter also discusses the impact of sleep on mental health and emotional wellbeing, highlighting that sleep disturbances can contribute to anxiety and depression, as well as impairing cognitive function and memory consolidation. Readers are encouraged to prioritize sleep as a vital component of overall health and wellbeing.

Mindfulness: The Key to Unlocking Your Full Potential

The concept of mindfulness and how it can help individuals unlock their full potential in various aspects of life, including personal and professional pursuits. It starts by defining mindfulness as the practice of being fully present and engaged in the current moment, without judgment or distraction.

It's then delves into the science behind mindfulness, explaining how it can help individuals regulate their emotions, reduce stress and anxiety, and improve cognitive function. It provides evidence-based research showing that mindfulness can improve brain function, enhance creativity, and improve decision-making skills.

Next, the chapter discusses how to practice mindfulness, providing practical guidance on how to incorporate mindfulness into daily life. It offers various techniques such as mindful breathing, body scan, and meditation, highlighting how each technique can help individuals cultivate greater awareness, clarity, and focus.

The chapter also explores how mindfulness can enhance personal relationships and communication skills, explaining how it can help individuals cultivate empathy, compassion, and understanding in their interactions with others. It also highlights how mindfulness can be applied in a professional context, such as enhancing leadership skills and decision-making abilities.

Furthermore, there are benefits of mindfulness in promoting physical health and well-being, highlighting how it can help individuals manage chronic pain, improve sleep quality, and reduce inflammation in the body.

Movement Matters: The Importance of Physical Activity for Health

"Movement Matters: The Importance of Physical Activity for Health" refers to the crucial role that regular physical activity plays in maintaining and promoting overall health and well-being.

Physical activity, which encompasses any form of bodily movement that results in energy expenditure, is essential for maintaining a healthy body weight, reducing the risk of chronic diseases, and promoting mental health. Despite these benefits, physical inactivity has become a major public health issue, with sedentary lifestyles and screen time on the rise.

Regular physical activity can improve cardiovascular health by reducing the risk of heart disease, stroke, and high blood pressure. It can also improve metabolic health by reducing the risk of type 2 diabetes, improving insulin sensitivity, and promoting healthy cholesterol levels. Physical activity is also essential for maintaining healthy bones and muscles, reducing the risk of osteoporosis and sarcopenia (muscle loss), and improving overall physical function and mobility.

In addition to physical health benefits, regular physical activity is also linked to improved mental health outcomes, such as reducing the risk of depression, anxiety, and stress. Physical activity can also improve cognitive function, including memory, attention, and executive function.

Overall, movement matters for our health and well-being. Incorporating regular physical activity into our daily routines is an important step towards promoting and maintaining a healthy lifestyle.

The Power of Connection: Social Support and Well-being

"The Power of Connection: Social Support and Well-being" refers to the significant role that social connections and support play in promoting and maintaining overall well-being. Social support encompasses emotional, informational, and practical assistance provided by individuals or groups within one's social network.

Research has consistently shown that individuals with strong social connections and support systems tend to have better physical and mental health outcomes. Strong social support has been linked to lower rates of depression, anxiety, and stress, and improved coping skills during times of stress or crisis.

Social support can come from a variety of sources, including family, friends, co-workers, religious or community groups, and online communities. It can take the form of emotional support, such as providing empathy and understanding during difficult times, or practical support, such as offering help with tasks or providing financial assistance.

Social support can also serve as a buffer against the negative effects of stress. People with strong social support systems may experience less stress and have a better ability to cope with stress when it does occur. Social support can also improve physical health outcomes by encouraging healthy behaviors, such as exercise, healthy eating, and regular medical check-ups.

Furthermore, social isolation and loneliness have been identified as significant risk factors for poor health outcomes, including depression, anxiety, cardiovascular disease, and even premature death. This highlights the importance of maintaining and strengthening social connections, especially as people age or experience significant life changes, such as retirement or the loss of a loved one.

Overall, the power of connection through social support is a crucial factor in promoting and maintaining overall well-being. By building and maintaining strong social connections, individuals can improve their physical and mental health outcomes, and better cope with the challenges of life.

Stress, Health, and Coping Strategies

"Stress, Health, and Coping Strategies" refers to the complex relationship between stress and physical and mental health, and the various strategies people use to cope with stress.

Stress is a natural response to challenges or demands in our environment. When we experience stress, our bodies release hormones such as adrenaline and cortisol, which trigger a range of physiological responses designed to help us cope with the stressor. However, when stress becomes chronic or overwhelming, it can have negative effects on our health, including increased risk of cardiovascular disease, depression, anxiety, and other health problems.

To cope with stress, people use a variety of strategies, both healthy and unhealthy. Healthy coping strategies include engaging in physical activity, practicing mindfulness or relaxation techniques, seeking social support, and engaging in hobbies or activities that provide a sense of purpose and enjoyment. Unhealthy coping strategies, on the other hand, can include excessive alcohol or drug use, overeating, or engaging in other self-destructive behaviors.

It is important to note that not all coping strategies are equally effective for everyone. What works for one person may not work for another, and individuals may need to experiment with different coping strategies to find what works best for them. In addition, effective coping strategies may change depending on the type and severity of stressor.

Effective coping strategies can help to reduce the negative effects of stress on physical and mental health. For example, physical activity can help to reduce stress and improve cardiovascular health, while mindfulness or relaxation techniques can help to reduce anxiety and improve overall well-being.

Overall, understanding the relationship between stress, health, and coping strategies is crucial for maintaining optimal health and well-being. By developing and using effective coping strategies, individuals can better manage stress and reduce its negative effects on their physical and mental health.

Balancing Act: The Connection Between Mental and Physical Health

"Balancing Act: The Connection Between Mental and Physical Health" refers to the intricate relationship between mental and physical health, and the impact they have on each other.

Physical and mental health are closely linked, with changes in one often impacting the other. For example, chronic physical illnesses such as diabetes, heart disease, or chronic pain, can significantly impact mental health, leading to depression, anxiety, and stress. Similarly, mental health conditions such as depression, anxiety, and post-traumatic stress disorder (PTSD) can have negative effects on physical health, leading to higher rates of cardiovascular disease, obesity, and other health problems.

There are several reasons why mental and physical health are so closely intertwined. One reason is that stress and other negative emotions can cause physical changes in the body, such as increased inflammation, higher blood pressure, and weakened immune function, which can contribute to the development of chronic diseases.

On the other hand, positive emotions such as joy, gratitude, and love, can have positive effects on physical health, including reducing inflammation and boosting immune function. Engaging in healthy behaviors such as regular exercise, healthy eating, and adequate sleep can also have positive effects on both physical and mental health.

To maintain a balance between physical and mental health, it is essential to prioritize both. This can involve seeking appropriate medical care for physical health concerns, such as managing chronic conditions or addressing injuries. It can also involve seeking appropriate mental health care, such as therapy or medication, for mental health concerns.

Additionally, practicing healthy behaviors such as engaging in regular physical activity, eating a healthy diet, getting adequate sleep, and managing stress through mindfulness, relaxation, or other techniques can also have positive effects on both physical and mental health.

Overall, the connection between mental and physical health underscores the importance of prioritizing both to achieve optimal health and well-being. By recognizing the interplay between the two and taking steps to address both, individuals can maintain a healthy balance and lead fulfilling lives.

Cultivating Healthy Habits: Sustainability Over Time

Cultivating Healthy Habits: Sustainability Over Time" refers to the importance of adopting and maintaining healthy habits that can be sustained over the long term.

Healthy habits can include a variety of behaviors, such as regular physical activity, healthy eating, getting adequate sleep, managing stress, and avoiding harmful behaviors such as smoking or excessive alcohol use. Adopting healthy habits can have a range of benefits for physical and mental health, including reduced risk of chronic diseases, improved mood, and increased energy and vitality.

However, developing healthy habits is not always easy, and it can be challenging to sustain these habits over time. Many people may experience setbacks or challenges in their efforts to adopt healthy habits, such as lack of motivation, difficulty finding time to exercise, or difficulty resisting unhealthy temptations.

To cultivate healthy habits that can be sustained over time, it is important to focus on making gradual, sustainable changes rather than attempting to make drastic changes all at once. This can involve setting realistic goals and breaking them down into smaller, more manageable steps. For example, rather than trying to completely overhaul your diet overnight, you might start by incorporating more fruits and vegetables into your meals and gradually reducing your intake of processed foods.

It is also important to find activities and behaviors that you enjoy and that fit into your lifestyle. This can help to increase motivation and make it more likely that you will stick with healthy habits over time. For example, if you enjoy hiking, you might incorporate more outdoor activities into your routine to increase physical activity levels.

Additionally, seeking support from others can be helpful in cultivating healthy habits over time. This might involve enlisting the help of a friend or family member to exercise with you, or joining a support group or online community focused on healthy living.

Overall, cultivating healthy habits that can be sustained over time requires patience, perseverance, and a willingness to adapt to changing circumstances. By focusing on making gradual, sustainable changes, finding enjoyable activities, and seeking support from others, individuals can increase the likelihood of successfully adopting and maintaining healthy habits over the long term.

Despite the many advances and breakthroughs, there are also challenges to overcome, such as the need to address disparities in access to healthcare and the potential ethical and social implications of new technologies.

Overall, the future of health holds great promise for improving health outcomes and quality of life, but it will require ongoing collaboration and innovation across healthcare providers, researchers, policymakers, and patients to realize this potential.

Your Personal Health Code: Putting it All Together.

Your Personal Health Code is a collection of guidelines, practices, and habits that you develop over time to promote your physical, mental, and emotional well-being. Putting it all together requires careful consideration and effort, but the benefits are well worth it. Here are some key elements to consider when developing your Personal Health Code:

Nutrition: Start by assessing your current eating habits and making changes to improve your overall nutrition. This may include eating a balanced diet with plenty of fruits, vegetables, lean proteins, and whole grains. You may also want to consider limiting processed foods, sugary drinks, and alcohol.

Exercise: Physical activity is crucial for maintaining good health. Develop an exercise routine that works for you, based on your fitness level, interests, and schedule. Aim for at least 150 minutes of moderate aerobic activity per week, as well as strength training exercises to build muscle and maintain bone density.

Sleep: Getting enough quality sleep is essential for good health. Aim for 7-9 hours of sleep per night, and establish a consistent sleep schedule. Avoid caffeine, alcohol, and electronics before bedtime, and create a relaxing sleep environment.

Stress management: Chronic stress can have a negative impact on your health. Develop strategies for managing stress, such as mindfulness, meditation, deep breathing, or yoga. Regular exercise can also help to reduce stress.

Relationships: Healthy relationships are important for emotional well-being. Cultivate meaningful connections with family, friends, and community members. Practice good communication, empathy, and active listening.

Mental health: Take care of your mental health by prioritizing self-care, seeking support when needed, and managing any mental health conditions. This may involve therapy, medication, or other treatments as recommended by your healthcare provider.

Preventive care: Regular check-ups, screenings, and preventive care can help you detect and manage health issues before they become more serious. Stay up-to-date on vaccinations, dental and vision exams, and screenings for conditions such as cancer, heart disease, and diabetes.

Remember, your Personal Health Code is unique to you. It may take some time to develop and refine your habits and practices, but the effort is worth it for the many benefits that come with good health. By prioritizing your well-being and taking a holistic approach to health, you can enjoy a happier, healthier life.

www.ingramcontent.com/pod-product-compliance
Lightning Source LLC
Chambersburg PA
CBHW061559250726
48657CB00021B/2339